CHILDREN IN CRISIS
Living after Chernobyl

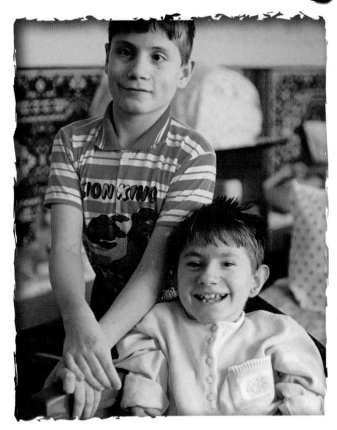

Ira's Story

Linda Walker

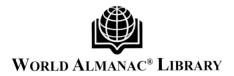

WORLD ALMANAC® LIBRARY

Please visit our web site at: www.worldalmanaclibrary.com
For a free color catalog describing World Almanac® Library's list of high-quality books and multimedia programs, call 1-800-848-2928 (USA) or 1-800-387-3178 (Canada). World Almanac® Library's fax: (414) 332-3567.

Library of Congress Cataloging-in-Publication Data

Walker, Linda.
    Living after Chernobyl: Ira's story / by Linda Walker.
      p. cm. — (Children in crisis)
    Includes bibliographical references and index.
    ISBN 0-8368-5957-X (lib. bdg.)
    1. Radiation injuries in children—Patients—Rehabilitation—Belarus. 2. Child health services—Belarus. 3. Chernobyl Nuclear Accident, Chornobyl§' Ukraine, 1986—Health aspects—Belarus.
I. Title. II. Children in crisis (Milwaukee, Wis.)
RJ384.W35   2005
618.92'9897—dc22
                                                2005046325

This North American edition first published in 2006 by
World Almanac® Library
A Member of the WRC Media Family of Companies
330 West Olive Street, Suite 100
Milwaukee, WI 53212 USA

This U.S. edition copyright © 2006 by World Almanac® Library. Original edition copyright © 2005 by ticktock Entertainment Ltd. First published in 2005 by ticktock Media Ltd, Unit 2, Orchard Business Centre, North Farm Road, Tunbridge Wells, Kent TN2 3XF, U.K.

World Almanac® Library editor: Alan Wachtel
World Almanac® Library managing editor: Valerie J. Weber
World Almanac® Library art direction: Tammy West
World Almanac® Library cover design and layout: Dave Kowalski
World Almanac® Library production: Jessica Morris

Photo credits: (t=top; b=bottom; l=left; r=right): Chernobyl Children's Project (UK) – Linda Walker: cover and pp. 1, 3, 5l, 7, 8, 9b, 11b, 11t, 12, 13t, 14, 15t, 16, 17, 18, 19b, 19t, 20, 21, 22, 23b, 23t, 24, 25b, 25t, 26b, 26t, 27, 28, 29b, 29t, 30, 31, 32, 33b, 33t, 34, 35b, 35t, 36, 37, 38–39, 40, 41b, 41t, 43b, 43t, 44, 45; CORBIS: 9t, 42; Getty images: 10; Magnum: 6b, 13b, 15b; Photos12: 5r.

Printed in the United States of America

1 2 3 4 5 6 7 8 9 09 08 07 06 05

The Interviewers

The interviews with Ira (the subject of the book) were conducted by Linda Walker, the national coordinator of the British charity Chernobyl Children's Project [CCP] (UK), and Liena Fedarchuk, who works as the director of CCP (UK)'s work in Gomel. CCP (UK) has been working in Belarus since 1995, helping children affected by the Chernobyl nuclear accident.

How Ira Was Chosen

Linda says: *"During my work in Belarus with CCP (UK), I have met many children who have suffered serious illnesses and disabilities and terrible hardships as a result of the 1986 Chernobyl disaster. I have known Ira since she was nine years old and chose her as the subject for this book because her severe disabilities and the limited life she has led have not dimmed her spirit."*

The Interview Process

The interviews held in November 2004 with Ira, her friends, teachers, and caregivers were carried out in Russian by Liena Fedarchuk. The interview texts were then translated into English. Linda Walker and the members of CCP (UK), as well as Ira's friends, caregivers, and teachers, have many memories of Ira's life and have helped to explain parts of her story that Ira does not herself remember.

CONTENTS

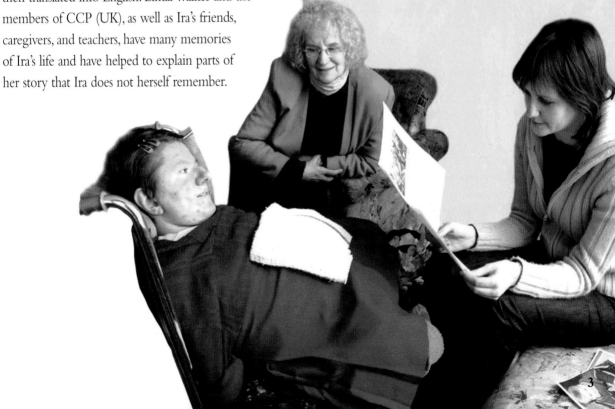

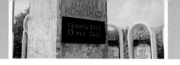

Introduction

In the early hours of Saturday, April 26, 1986, the world's worst nuclear accident took place at the Chernobyl power station in Ukraine. Over the following days, a disaster unfolded that had terrible, long-term consequences for the people of Ukraine, Belarus, and western Russia.

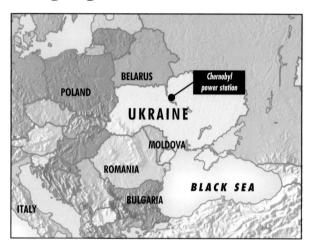

Chernobyl is 62 miles (100 kilometers) north of Ukraine's capital, Kiev, and 7.5 miles (12 km) south of its border with Belarus.

A NIGHTMARE SITUATION

At the time of the Chernobyl accident, Ukraine, Belarus, and Russia were part of the Soviet Union. Along with many other Soviet republics, Ukraine relied on nuclear power to supply a significant amount of its electricity. On the night of April 26, 1986, an inexperienced operating crew carried out a potentially dangerous safety check on the cooling system of the Unit 4 reactor at the Chernobyl power station. During the test, a sudden power surge caused the reactor to reach one hundred times its normal power in a matter of seconds. The emergency shutdown failed, and then, the worst thing possible happened—the crew lost control of the reactor.

Power levels and temperatures inside the reactor rose, causing a massive explosion. The reactor building's 1,100-ton (1,000-metric ton) sealing cap was blown off, and a lethal shower of radioactive material was launched 5,000 feet (1,500 meters) into the air. As temperatures inside the reactor soared to more than 3,600° Fahrenheit (2,000° Celsius), the reactor's protective graphite covering ignited, creating a poisonous, blazing inferno.

THE FIRST CHERNOBYL VICTIMS

In the days that followed the accident, hundreds of soldiers and workers from the power station's fire and operating crews were drafted to fight the blaze. Both the power-station management and the Soviet authorities, however, were unprepared for a disaster of this magnitude, and the workers were not issued any breathing apparatus or protective clothing. Some of the firefighters received doses of radiation up to thirteen thousand times higher than the maximum annual amount deemed safe by the European Union for people who live near a nuclear power plant. Unable to get any medical help, many of these workers fell ill, and some died within weeks of the accident.

For ten days, the fire continued to burn, propelling radioactive particles into the atmosphere. Finally, on May 6, the blaze was extinguished, and the radioactive emissions were brought under control.

A SECRET DISASTER

As with many aspects of life in the Soviet Union, the Chernobyl disaster was immediately shrouded in secrecy. The Soviet authorities were afraid of creating a panic and hoped to keep this huge failure in their nuclear program a secret. Officials in Moscow insisted there had only been a small accident and that there was no threat to the health of the population. The reluctance of the Soviet authorities to admit the scale of the disaster caused serious delays in advising people about how to protect themselves in the aftermath of the accident.

This memorial in Bragin, Belarus, is dedicated to one of the firefighters who died as a result of the Chernobyl accident.

CHERNOBYL TIME LINE

12/21/83: Chernobyl reactor Unit 4 goes on-line ahead of schedule but with many safety tests not completed.

4/26/86: Chernobyl reactor Unit 4 runs out of control during a safety test and explodes.

4/26/86–5/5/86: Wind and rain spread radiation over Ukraine, Belarus, western Russia, and parts of Europe. Eighteen hundred helicopter flights deposit 5,500 tons (5,000 metric tons) of lead and sand onto the burning reactor to smother the fire and absorb the radiation.

4/28/86: A Danish nuclear research laboratory announces there has been a major accident at Chernobyl. Government-run Moscow TV tells the people of the Soviet Union that an accident has occurred at Chernobyl. No details are given.

Up to 5/6/86: The reactor is cooled by liquid nitrogen pumped beneath it. The fire is extinguished. Radioactive releases stop.

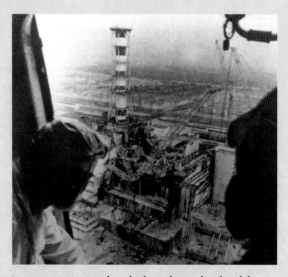

A power station worker checks radiation levels while flying over the destroyed Unit 4 reactor in a helicopter in May 1986.

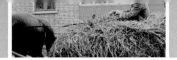

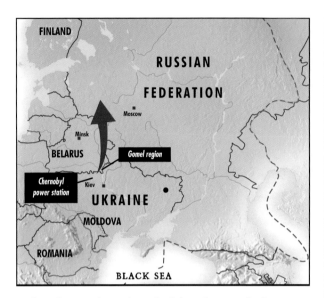

The red arrow shows the path of the radioactive cloud as winds carried it north in the first few days after the accident.

WHAT IS NUCLEAR POWER?

Nuclear power has been used to produce electricity since the 1950s. The power is produced by a process called nuclear fission. In nuclear fission, a chain reaction is created in which radioactive atoms shoot out neutrons that split other atoms. This process produces energy in the form of heat.

Inside a nuclear reactor, fuel rods made from uranium (a radioactive element) are placed in the reactor's core. The rods are close enough for their neutrons to strike each other. As the atoms in the fuel rods split apart, the rods heat up, raising the temperature of the cooling water around them, which then turns to steam. The steam powers turbines, which spin to produce electricity.

EVACUATIONS

On April 27, thirty-six hours after the accident, 45,000 people were evacuated from Pripyat, a town just about 2 miles (3 km) from Chernobyl. Over the next ten days, a 19-mile (30-km) exclusion zone was set up around the power station, and a further 130,000 people were evacuated from their homes in seventy-six towns and villages.

IN THE PATH OF THE CLOUD

To the north of Ukraine lies Belarus, a beautiful country of large forests, marshlands, lakes, rivers, and farms. In the days following the accident, winds carried huge clouds of radioactive particles north, depositing an estimated 70 percent of the Chernobyl fallout onto Belarus. Localized heavy rain showers resulted in radioactive "hot spots" hundreds of miles from the plant. Some areas, such as Gomel, in southern Belarus, became as severely contaminated as pieces of land in the immediate vicinity of the Chernobyl reactor.

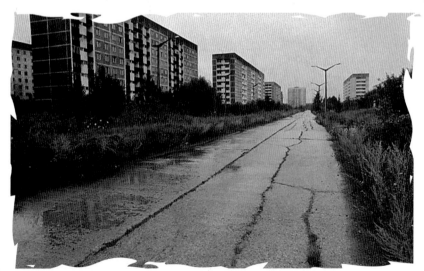

The town of Pripyat was built to house Chernobyl workers and their families. Today, it is still deserted because of dangerous levels of radiation.

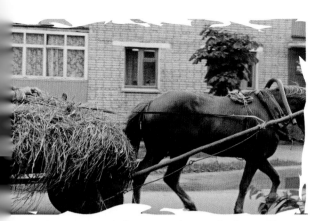

Even today, many people living in rural areas of Belarus still use a horse-drawn cart as their main form of transportation.

LIVING FROM THE LAND

Belarus has a population of about 10 million people and is one of the poorest countries in Europe. Belarussian people live on low incomes (the average annual income is U.S. $1,300), and many rely on food they grow or produce themselves. Following the Chernobyl disaster, Belarussians continued to consume home-grown vegetables, wild berries, fungi, and milk from cows that had eaten contaminated grass. They were unaware that they were eating and drinking radioactive substances. It would be many weeks before the authorities warned them that food produced around their homes could be dangerously contaminated.

EXTENDING THE DANGER ZONE

Over time, many people came to believe that the radioactive contamination simply stopped at the border of the exclusion zone. It was not until 1989 that *Pravda* (the main Soviet newspaper) published accurate maps of the contaminated area.

The maps showed that some areas 185 miles (300 km) to the north of the Chernobyl plant were equally contaminated as those inside the exclusion zone. A second series of evacuations began.

CHERNOBYL TIME LINE

11/15/86: A 300,000-ton (272,000-metric ton) reinforced concrete structure, built to contain reactor Unit 4, is completed.

November 1986: Chernobyl reactors Unit 1 and Unit 2 return to operation.

December 1987: Reactor Unit 3, which was damaged by the explosion, is repaired and put back in operation.

4/20/89: The Soviet government halts construction work on Chernobyl reactors Unit 5 and Unit 6.

1991: The Soviet Union falls, and Ukraine, Belarus, and Russia become independent countries, inheriting all the economic, social, and health problems caused by the Chernobyl disaster.

1993: A thyroid center is established in Gomel by the Otto Hug Strahleninstitut of Munich, Germany.

7/5/00: The G7 countries, the European Union (EU), and Ukraine pledge U.S. $715 million to build a new shelter for reactor Unit 4.

12/12/00: The Chernobyl nuclear power station is closed down.

April 2001: At the "Fifteen Years after Chernobyl Accident—Lessons Learned" conference in Kiev, a direct link between the accident and thyroid cancer in children is internationally recognized.

2001: Scientists from around the world call for further research into links between the Chernobyl accident, genetic abnormalities, and medical conditions such as cancer.

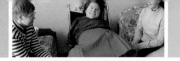

CHAPTER ONE: A Chernobyl Baby

Following the Chernobyl accident, there has been a significant increase in the number of people in parts of Belarus, Ukraine, and Russia suffering from serious illnesses. Many of the people worst affected are children. Most experts now agree that the increase in conditions such as cancer, heart disease, and diabetes is linked to the exposure to radiation that the people of the Chernobyl region suffered. Exposure to radiation also carries another hidden cost. In the areas contaminated by the radioactive fallout, the number of babies born with physical or mental disabilities has risen.

LINDA WALKER SAYS:

"Ira was born just two years after the Chernobyl disaster, in a village called Tihinichi, in the north of the Gomel Region. Gomel is the most contaminated part of Belarus, and there has been an estimated 80 percent rise in the number

In January 2005, Linda Walker visited Ira at Rechitsa Boarding School in Gomel, Belarus. Ira has lived at Rechitsa since 2003.

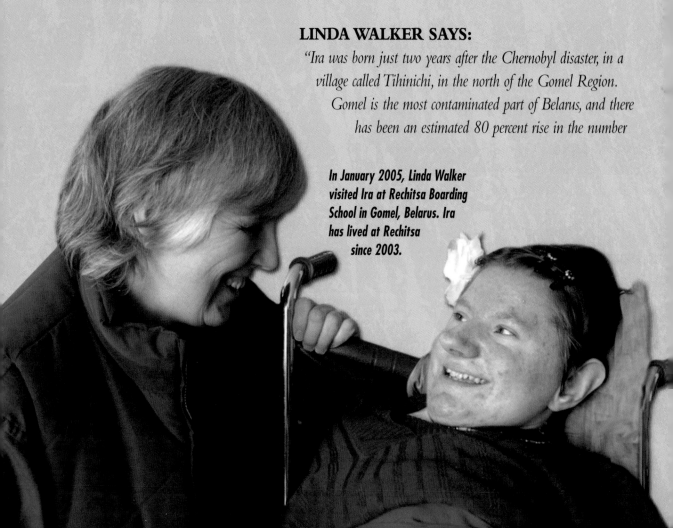

of children born with disabilities in this area since the Chernobyl accident.

Ira was born with damage to all her limbs: Her legs are very short and her feet twist inward; her arms are also short, and her left hand twists outward. Her disabilities were very likely caused by her mother's exposure to radiation.

Members of Chernobyl Children's Project [CCP] (UK) first met Ira when she was nine years old. When we toured the cots full of disabled children on our visits to the Zhuravichi Children's Home in Gomel, Ira would always have a bright smile for us. However, it would be two years before we learned the full extent of how intelligent she was.

For eleven years, Ira spent almost all her time lying in a cot with nothing to do and little or no stimulation. But Ira has huge strength of character—all she needed was to be given a chance."

RADIATION AND CANCER

Cancers form when the body's cells begin to multiply abnormally, producing cell masses called tumors. Nuclear radiation is carcinogenic, meaning it increases the chances of the body's cells behaving in this way. Since the Chernobyl accident, doctors in the contaminated regions have reported an increase in the number of brain tumors, cases of leukemia, and other cancers.

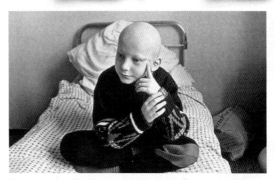

This young boy has been receiving chemotherapy treatment for cancer. One side effect of the treatment is hair loss.

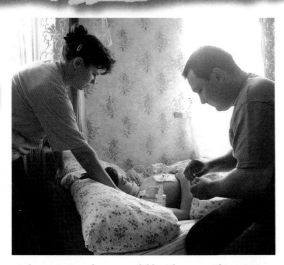

A doctor in Gomel treats a child with cancer. The majority of thyroid cancer sufferers are children and young people.

THYROID CANCER

In the years after the accident, there has been a dramatic increase in the incidence of thyroid cancer across Belarus. The thyroid gland, which is located in the neck, takes in and stores the iodine that is needed by the body. During the Chernobyl accident, radioactive iodine was released into the atmosphere. This iodine was taken in by children's thyroid glands and stored, eventually causing cancer. Thyroid cancer is normally treated successfully, often by the surgical removal of the thyroid gland, which leaves patients requiring medication for the rest of their lives.

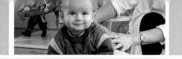

"When Ira was born with such severe disabilities, her mother must have been deeply shocked. In the Soviet Union at the time when Ira was born, attitudes towards children with disabilities were very much as they were in Britain in Victorian times. Children, like Soviet society, were supposed to be perfect. If they had obvious disabilities they were a source of deep embarrassment, and fathers, in particular, were not willing to bring up a disabled child as part of their family.

Doctors normally advised the mothers of even mildly disabled babies to give their children away. In Ira's case, the doctors may have genuinely believed that she would not survive for long, as she must have been very tiny and weak. The mother of an autistic child born fourteen years ago puts it like this, 'When my son was born I had two choices. I could put him in an institution and throw his life away. Or I could keep him with me and throw my life away.' There were no other options available to desperate mothers at that time.

Today, there are many associations of parents in Belarus helping each other to support their disabled children. They persuade the government to do more to help and work with foreign partners. Sixteen years ago, there were no such associations and there would have been nowhere for Ira's mother to turn for help if she had considered trying to keep her baby.

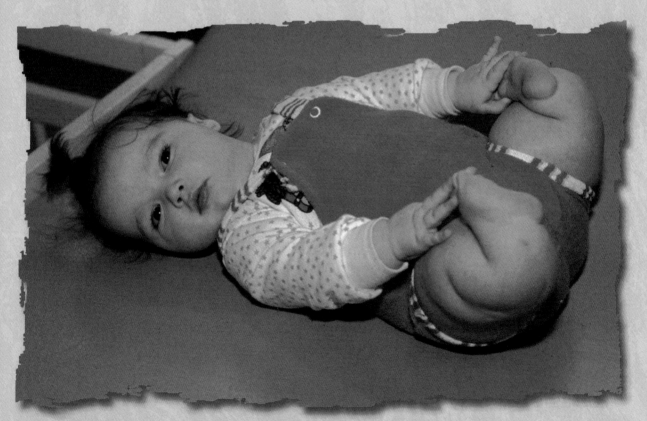

This little girl was born with deformities to her legs and feet. She was born in Belarus six years after the Chernobyl accident—like Ira, in Belarus. There are no existing photographs of Ira as a baby or young child.

So Ira was given away to the Abandoned Babies' Home in Gomel. Natalia, one of Ira's caregivers at the Zhuravichi Children's Home (where Ira went to live when she was four years old), told us, 'Ira's family and parents never came to visit her and never contacted the orphanage about her. We think the mother rejected her in the maternity hospital because Ira was born very disabled.'"

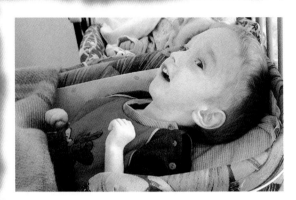

This little boy at the Abandoned Babies' Home was born with hydrocephalus, an accumulation of fluid in the brain that makes the head enlarge. Hydrocephalus can cause mental disabilities.

BIRTH DEFECTS

Levels of radiation that are too low to kill human cells can still cause damage by disrupting the cells' DNA—the genetic material stored in cells that determines what a person will be like as he or she grows. Radiation damage to egg or sperm cells can lead to abnormalities in children that are conceived not just in the current generation but also in future generations. If a woman is exposed to radiation during pregnancy, the fetus she is carrying may die or the baby may be born with disabilities.

THE ABANDONED BABIES' HOME

Today, more than one hundred babies and young children still live at the Abandoned Babies' Home in Gomel. About forty of these children have disabilities such as Down Syndrome, autism, cerebral palsy, spina bifida, hydrocephalus, microcephaly, missing limbs, or severe learning disabilities.

Most of the babies at the home who do not have a disability were born to young, single mothers or families that are too poor to keep them. These children are likely to be adopted either in Belarus or abroad, but it is very rare for a child with a disability to be adopted or even put in foster care.

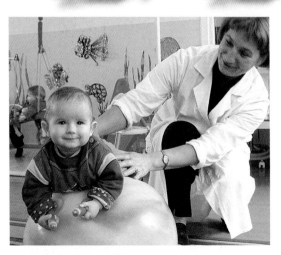

With overseas help, conditions at the Abandoned Babies' Home have improved since the 1980s. It has become a bright, better-equipped facility with professionally trained staff.

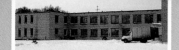

CHAPTER TWO: Life at Zhuravichi

After four years at the Abandoned Babies' Home, Ira was moved to the Zhuravichi Children's Home, a huge institution hidden deep in the Gomel countryside. Over two hundred children, with a wide range of physical and mental disabilities among them, were living at Zhuravichi.

LINDA WALKER SAYS:

"It took Chernobyl Children's Project (UK) several months to discover where the most disabled children were sent when they left the baby home in Gomel.

When we first visited Zhuravichi, most of the rooms were bare and gloomy, and it was quite a depressing place. The children were kept clean, dressed, and fed, but for many of them, especially the fifty who were living in cots, that was about it. There were very few toys, wheelchairs, or disability aids and no bean bags or comfy mats where children from the cots could spend some time out of bed.

For intelligent children who could not walk, life was especially bleak at Zhuravichi. Their physical

disabilities meant they were regarded as being unable to learn. They had very little to occupy their time and no opportunities to learn to read.

Ira had been put into a large room with twenty very disabled children, the majority of whom had severe learning difficulties as well as their physical problems. All the children, including Ira, spent their days just lying in their cots."

IRA SAYS:

"I can't remember much about my life when I used to lie in the cot all the time. I do remember hearing children crying a lot and one caregiver who was very kind

When Ira went to live in the Zhuravichi Children's Home in 1992, almost no one in Belarus knew that such homes existed.

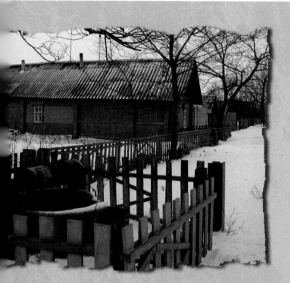

This small, wooden house is located in Tihinichi, the village where Ira was born. Many poorer homes in Belarus had no running water, and families had to draw their water from a well.

and friendly, but I have forgotten her name. She used to talk to me about her family, and I wished she was my mom. I liked it when I had a bath, the feeling of warm water, and being sleepy afterward."

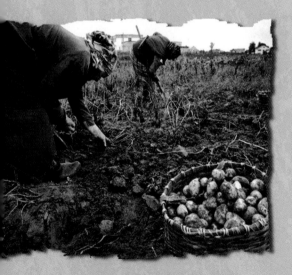

In the Belarussian village of Maiski, women harvest potatoes grown close to the exclusion zone. Poor families had no option but to continue to eat food they had grown in contaminated soil.

A COUNTRY IN CRISIS

With the break-up of the Soviet Union in 1991, the newly independent government of Belarus was left to manage the aftermath of the Chernobyl disaster on its own. The authorities struggled to cope with the costly projects of moving people away from the most contaminated areas, building housing accommodations for these evacuees, and providing uncontaminated food and proper health care for people from affected areas.

• Life for people in Belarus was much harder after the Chernobyl accident. People lived with the constant anxiety that they or their children would become sick from exposure to radiation.

• Families evacuated from contaminated areas were often moved from country villages to specially built high-rise apartment buildings in the cities.

• For many families, it was a great strain to leave behind family graves that were in the exclusion zone. In Belarus, it is customary for people to live near where their parents and grandparents are buried.

• People who had to resettle in new places found it hard to fit in and find jobs in the cities to which they moved. They also lived with the stigma of having been exposed to radiation, which many people thought was contagious.

• Children from affected areas were bullied in their new schools and called "Chernobyls."

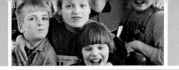
LINDA WALKER SAYS:

"In the early 1990s, institutions such as Zhuravichi were a low priority for the government of Belarus. The budget of an orphanage like Zhuravichi provided for the staff salaries, heating, simple food, and basic clothes for the children, but very little else. The caregivers at the orphanage worked hard to look after the children, but they had to work long hours and were poorly paid. They had no time or energy to give the children the attention they craved. Some of the more capable children were trained in craft skills, but most of the children did not have any lessons.

We would walk around the cot rooms, moving sadly from bed to bed. Some of the children had twisted limbs, some were blind, a few had severe breathing problems. From some of the children we could get a smile or even giggles by fussing over them. Others looked at us quite blankly, and some were frightened by the presence of strangers.

It was always a pleasure to get to Ira's bed and see her smile as soon as we spoke to her. Like all the children living in the cots, Ira needed to wear a nappie [diaper]. Proper nappies, either cloth or disposable, were seldom available, so the children often had to wear pieces of cloth which were not very absorbent.

When Ira was quite small, probably nine years old, one of the caregivers told us that she was so delicate, it caused her pain to have her clothes changed or to be taken for a bath. Ira does not remember this, and as she grew bigger, she became stronger and healthier and could be lifted and moved without any problems."

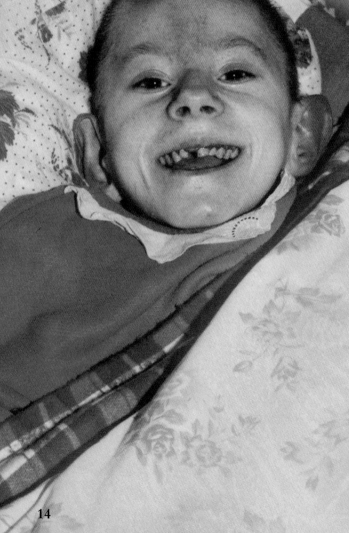

Shown lying in her cot at Zhuravichi, Ira is about nine years old in this picture.

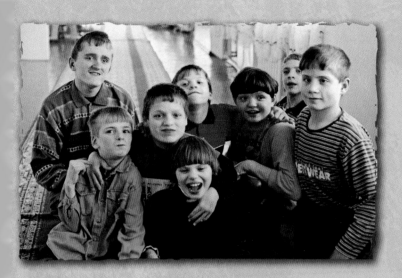

This picture of a group of the Zhuravichi children was taken in 1998. Ira's best friend at Zhuravichi, Vova, is shown on the far right of the photograph.

HOW LONG WILL THE CONTAMINATION LAST?

The most significant radionuclides released at Chernobyl were iodine-131, cesium-137, and strontium-90. Radionuclides decay at different rates. For example, eight days after the accident, the level of radioactivity of the iodine-131 that was released had already halved. This is called the nuclide's "half-life." After another eight days, the amount halved again to leave a quarter of the original dose. Nearly twenty years later, the radioactivity levels of iodine-131 are now tiny. Cesium-137 and strontium-90, however, have half-lives of thirty years. It will take more than three hundred years for the levels of radioactivity to reach safer levels. Cesium-137 accumulates in the body's muscle tissue, while strontium-90 accumulates in bones.

THE DECONTAMINATION PLAN

At first, it was believed that it would be possible to "clean up" the contaminated areas close to the Chernobyl power station. The Soviet authorities drafted eight hundred thousand "liquidators," who worked for periods of up to six months. They scraped the topsoil from areas such as school playgrounds, washed the roofs and walls of buildings, and even demolished contaminated houses. Their work, however, did not achieve its goal. The towns and villages in the exclusion zone remained seriously contaminated. The Russian, Ukrainian, and Belarussian authorities say that, to date, twenty-five thousand of the liquidators have died from radiation-related illnesses.

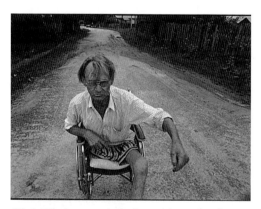

Nikolai Yanchen was drafted to work as a liquidator. He lost his right leg to cancer and now lives in a small village near the 19-mile (30-km) exclusion zone.

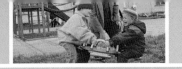

GLENDA NORRIS SAYS:

"I spent two months as a CCP (UK) volunteer at Zhuravichi in 1998. Most of my time was devoted to getting children out of the cots and giving them the chance to move around a little.

Ira was not allowed to spend much time out of her cot, so I tried to think of ways to entertain her where she was. She was always pleased to see me, but I don't speak Russian so I could not communicate with her much. I had a tapestry of the alphabet—British, not Russian—and I hung that above her bed, and taught her the first few letters. Within a week she had learned most of the alphabet. She was so anxious to learn and so happy when I praised her skill. It was a joy to work with her."

This picture shows Ira at eleven years old with Glenda Norris, who volunteered with CCP (UK) from 1998 to 2000 and worked with Ira at Zhuravichi.

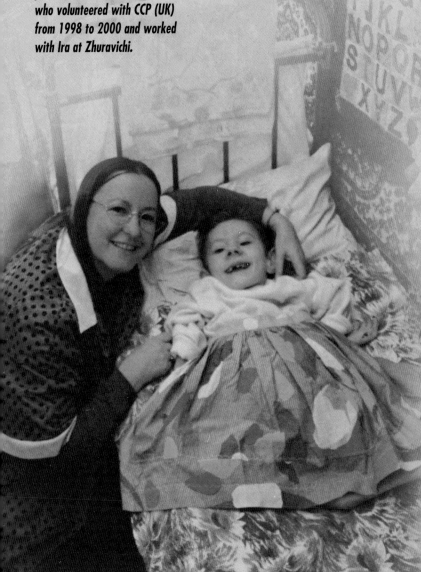

IRA SAYS:

"It was always a special day when visitors came. The caregivers would make sure everyone was ready for the visit. If they suggested that I should wear a pretty dress, I was always very happy. Some days we had to wait hours before the visitors came to our room. When they came to my cot, I always felt very excited. I knew Mags and Linda best. They would say, 'Kraseeva' (beautiful) and I thought, 'They mean me!'

Glenda came to see me nearly every day when she was staying at Zhuravichi. After a while, she put a big cloth on the wall with letters on it. She taught me a few letters every day, and I would lie in bed looking at them and trying to remember them."

MAGS WHITING SAYS:

"Ira had always been special to me. She was the same age as my granddaughter, and one Christmas, when Ira was nine, I wrote a poem about her comparing Stephanie's happy, busy Christmas with the lonely time Ira would have. On every visit to Zhuravichi, I looked forward to seeing Ira with her radiant smile. But I thought, perhaps, she was happy because she did not understand very much.

Then, one day, Glenda Norris took Linda Walker and me to Ira's cot and said, 'Look what she can do!' With a smile from ear to ear, Ira read for us, 'ay, bee, cee, dee, ...,' almost all the way through the alphabet. I told her how clever she was. Then I turned away so she would not see the tears in my eyes."

Mags Whiting is a trustee of Chernobyl Children's Project (UK).

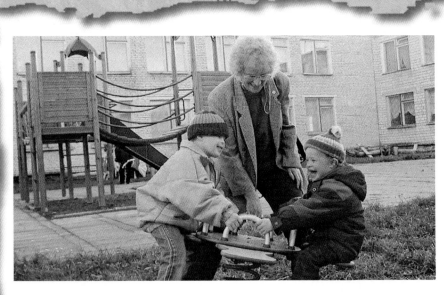

Mags Whiting plays with children in the Zhuravichi playground, which was built by CCP (UK) in 2001.

A CLOSED INSTITUTION

During the Soviet era, Zhuravichi was a closed institution, and no one was allowed to visit the children who lived there. When Ira first went to live at Zhuravichi in 1992, the home had a staff of two hundred, including cleaners, cooks, maintenance staff, and caregivers. Most of the caregivers, however, were untrained, and many did not even have a particular desire to work with children. They were local people, and there were few other jobs for them nearby.

ZHURAVICHI TODAY

In the past ten years, with the support of foreign partners and three Polish nuns who have lived at the home for more than six years, the Zhuravichi staff have transformed the children's environment. The home now has many toys and mobility aids, a physical-therapy room, a playground that is accessible to disabled children, and bathrooms with new toilets. The staff have been trained properly, and there are lessons and summer vacations for the children.

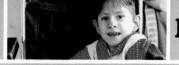

LINDA WALKER SAYS:

"When Ira's friends from the UK realized what a bright child she was, it seemed all the more tragic that she should be condemned to lie in a cot all day.

Ira is being pushed in a wheelchair by Tanya, another one of the girls at Zhuravichi. This picture was taken the first year Ira was put in a wheelchair.

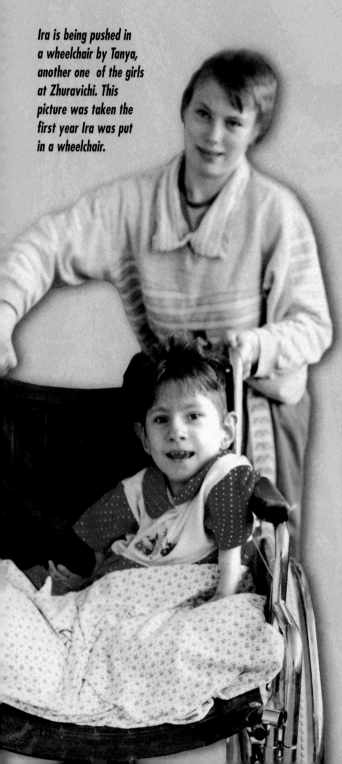

In 1999, CCP (UK) brought wheelchairs to Zhuravichi, and Ira was able to sit up for the first time in her life.

From her cot, Ira had seen nothing but a white ceiling. Once she was in the wheelchair, she could spend a few hours every day watching and talking to the people around her. However, Ira still only had tantalizing glimpses of the sky and the tops of trees through the high windows in her room. So, one warm summer day, Ira was taken outside for the first time."

IRA SAYS:

"When I was first taken out of my cot and placed in a wheelchair I was frightened. It felt so strange to be upright without a caregiver holding on to me. Once I realized I was safe, I felt very excited to be able to see all around me. Instead of having a quick look around as I was carried to the bath, I was able to look for as long as I liked at everything in my room. I could even sit in the corridor and watch children from other rooms coming and going for lunch or going to lessons.

Some days were special because we celebrated birthdays. We would all go to the gym, and some of the children would sing. We had sweets to eat and then we would have a dance. It was wonderful!

The first time I went outside, Vova [Ira's best friend at Zhuravichi] pushed me, and we went out into the garden. The sun was bright and hot, so we went to sit under the trees. I saw the cows in the field nearby, and I heard some birds

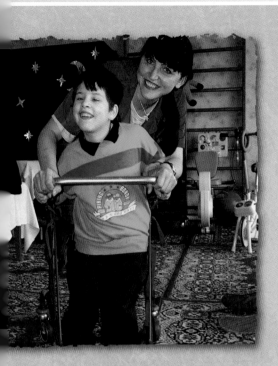

Luba, the physical therapist at Zhuravichi, tries some new equipment with Stas. Occupational therapists and physical therapists from Britain educated the caregivers at Zhuravichi about how to use mobility aids such as walking frames.

singing. I watched the children playing and felt the fresh air on my face."

LINDA WALKER SAYS:

"In the Spring of 2001, a CCP (UK) aid convoy delivered a variety of walking frames and special seats to Zhuravichi. These had all been donated by schools and hospitals in the UK, in some cases because they had acquired more modern equipment. A team of therapists from Devon spent several days at Zhuravichi. They fitted the physically disabled children into the most appropriate seats and showed the staff how to use the mobility aids."

CONTAMINATED BELARUS

For many of the most severely disabled Zhuravichi children, 1999 was the first year in their lives they were able to go outside. While they enjoyed the sunshine and "fresh" air, the environment around Zhuravichi was still badly contaminated by radioactive fallout thirteen years after the Chernobyl accident.

• People living in many villages in the Gomel region received more radiation within three to four years after the accident than is safe to receive over a lifetime. It has been estimated that southern Belarus was exposed to radioactivity ninety times greater than that released by the Hiroshima atomic bomb.

• In 1986, the average life expectancy in Belarus was 72.6 years. By 2000, it had dropped to 67.6 years.

• By 2000, the air was considered safe, but dust lifted by plowing or wind erosion could put radiation back into the air at any time.

• One-fourth of the farmland and one-fifth of the forests in Belarus were poisoned by radioactive contamination.

• Some areas are contaminated with the element plutonium, which has a half-life of twenty-four thousand years.

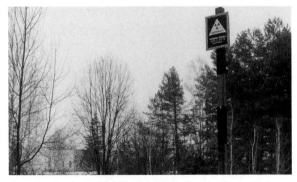

This is a forest area inside the exclusion zone. Summer forest fires can still spread radiation.

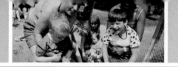

CHAPTER THREE: Dreams and New Goals

Most of the children at Zhuravichi had never been on vacation or even been outside the grounds of the orphanage. Chernobyl Children's Project (UK) organized a trip in Belarus for as many of them as possible.

LINDA WALKER SAYS:

"A few of the children from Zhuravichi had been to Italy to stay with families, but rather than take a few more abroad, we decided it would be best to try to arrange a holiday [vacation] in Belarus for as many children as possible. We found a sanatorium, or holiday camp, in a clean part of the country, where the director was willing to accept disabled children, and we persuaded the local authority to pay part of the cost. Raisa Ivanovna, the director at Zhuravichi, was asked to choose about eighty children who would get the most benefit from a holiday.

Unfortunately, Ira was not one of the children selected to go to the holiday camp. Doctors who visited Zhuravichi said she was too delicate and it would be too risky for her to travel.

When her friends set off for camp, Ira dreamed of going to the sanatorium holiday with them.

Ludmilla Markovna is a teacher at Zhuravichi. During the interviews for this book, Ludmilla told us, 'All the children live on

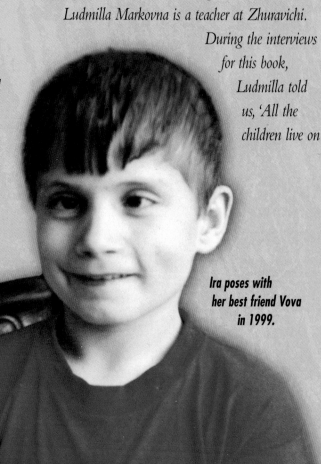

Ira poses with her best friend Vova in 1999.

their memories of the sanatorium all the year round. They enjoy it and often talk about it. They want to go to sanatorium holidays as they make new contacts and have so many new experiences. It is like a window into real life.'"

IRA SAYS:

"I felt upset when my friends and all the other children went to the holiday camp in the summer each year. There were lots of other children left behind, but most of them could not talk, so it was very lonely. I especially missed Vova.

I tried not to think about it and to just be happy talking to the caregivers, but I kept wondering what Vova and the other children were doing and wishing I could be there, too.

When Vova came back from the camp, he talked to me a lot about all the things he had been doing and how much he liked the volunteers who played with the children."

A VACATION FROM CONTAMINATION

Zhuravichi children began taking vacations in 1998 and have continued every summer. About seventy children from Zhuravichi travel from the eastern edge of Belarus to a beautiful area near the Polish border. Neman Sanatorium, or vacation camp, is in a part of Belarus untouched by the radiation from Chernobyl. CCP (UK) raises money to pay for extra food for the children and outings, and it arranges the transportation. About twenty volunteers fly from Britain to Belarus to work at the camp alongside the caregivers from Zhuravichi.

THREE WEEKS OF FUN

For three weeks at the sanatorium, the children from Zhuravichi paint; make masks, models, and puppets; perform puppet shows; and participate in storytelling and musical sessions. Some of the children play basketball or soccer, take part in races, and play catch. Every evening, there is either a dance or a film. Dances are a favorite activity, and the children who cannot walk love to be twirled around in their wheelchairs.

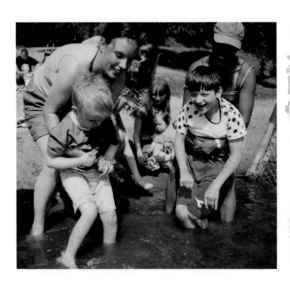

A variety of activities are organized so that every child can take part.

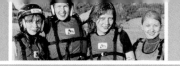

IRA SAYS:

"One day Linda came to visit. Vova and I were taken in a minibus to Gomel with one of my caregivers. We went to a nice house where Liena, Sasha, and Greesha were living. They all used to live at Zhuravichi, and they have disabilities, too. They were very nice to us. They gave us lots of good things to eat, and we watched television with them. We stayed there for a night and then a doctor came to see us the next day. The doctor was very nice and friendly and asked me lots of questions, which Vova helped me answer because I felt quite shy. Then we went back to Zhuravichi. I thought about the visit for days.

Linda came to see me again soon afterward. I recited a poem for the visitors that I had learned with Vova. Then Linda said something to Raisa Ivanovna, our director. The interpreter told me that in the summer [2002] I would be going to the vacation camp. I could not believe it, and I almost cried.

I was so excited the first time I went to the camp, I could not sleep the night before. We all got into the bus very early in the morning and set off with everyone, very noisy and happy. It was a long journey and so much to see! I looked out of the window most of the time at the forests and fields, houses and farms, cows and horses.

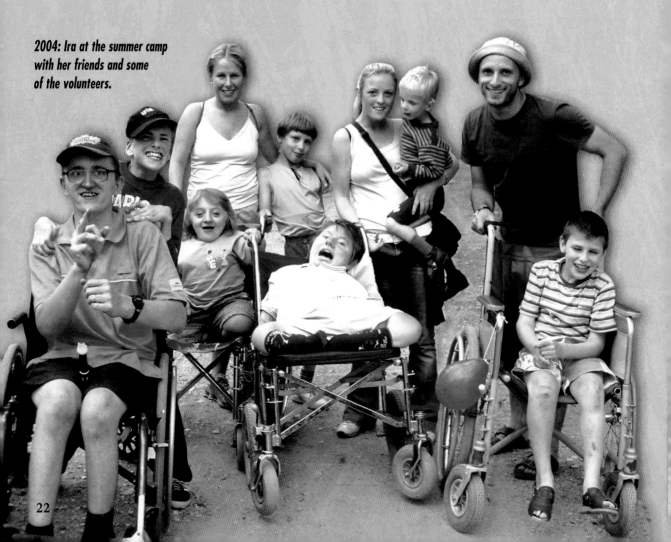

2004: Ira at the summer camp with her friends and some of the volunteers.

We went through Minsk, our capital city. It was huge and very beautiful and full of cars. I got tired from sitting up for so long, so I was able to lie down across the seats and sleep. Ludmilla Markovna looked after me on the journey and at the camp. She is very nice and kind.

It was nearly the end of the day when we got to the holiday camp. It was beautiful, lots of grass and trees. The British people were there to meet us, and we all went inside for something to eat and drink. Then we went to bed early because we were all so tired."

THE BENEFIT OF VACATIONS ABROAD

In 1991, doctors in Belarus appealed to the world for help in providing clean-air vacations for the children of their country. Since then, charities have arranged for many thousands of children to travel from Belarus to enjoy a few weeks of uncontaminated food, fresh air, relaxation, and fun. The children stay with families in Italy, Spain, Germany, France, the Netherlands, the United States, Canada, Britain, Ireland, and Wales. Some young children are accompanied by their mothers.

Many adults and children in the contaminated areas suffer from a variety of infections due to weakened immune systems.

Doctors say that just four weeks in a clean environment can help the children stay healthy or recover completely from illness. The vacations make a great difference to the children's immune systems and remove the build-up of radioactive substances from their bodies.

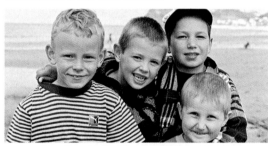

Max, who is from England (center), visits with his friends from Belarus, Maxim, Andrei, and Vadim, who are all in remission from cancer.

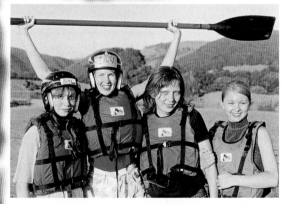

On a respite vacation in Wales in 2000, interpreter Natalia (second from left) poses with Youlia, Natasha, and Inna.

A PSYCHOLOGICAL BOOST

Many of the Belarussian children who go on vacations abroad are in remission after treatment for cancer. Others have had operations or have chronic illnesses. Some simply live in the more contaminated villages in the south and east of Belarus. Vacations provide a boost to the health of these children and teenagers and are also of psychological importance. The children return to Belarus feeling stronger and happier, with memories and photos of new experiences and friends.

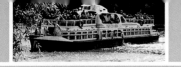

Living After Chernobyl

IRA SAYS:

"The food at the camp was nice, and we were often given fruit and sweets. The weather was lovely, the sun was shining nearly every day, and we were outside most of the time. It was good just to sit outside under the trees.

I liked all the English volunteers, especially Laura and Glenda. They took me for walks through the forest and down by the river. I watched the other children play and I really enjoyed watching concerts and going to the dances. I went for treatment and massage, too, and that made me feel better.

What I liked best of all was playing boogie-woogie OK [the Belarussian version of the hokey-pokey]. It was so good to be part of a big group, with everyone singing and laughing and Vova pushing me backward and forward in my wheelchair."

GLENDA TRACEY SAYS:

"When I worked as a volunteer at the holiday camp, my first impression of Ira was one of sadness, but by the end of the holiday all I had for her was love. She gains so much happiness by watching the other children enjoying themselves—it shows in her smile and eyes.

I remember taking her for a walk in her wheelchair for the first time over rough ground. She was not too sure, so we took a strap from a suitcase and made a safety belt across the chair—then she was up for exploring the grounds of the sanatorium and many other new experiences. The first time that Ira spoke to me she just came out with the words "cheeky monkey," an expression that I had been saying to her. After this, she would say it often, and start to laugh!"

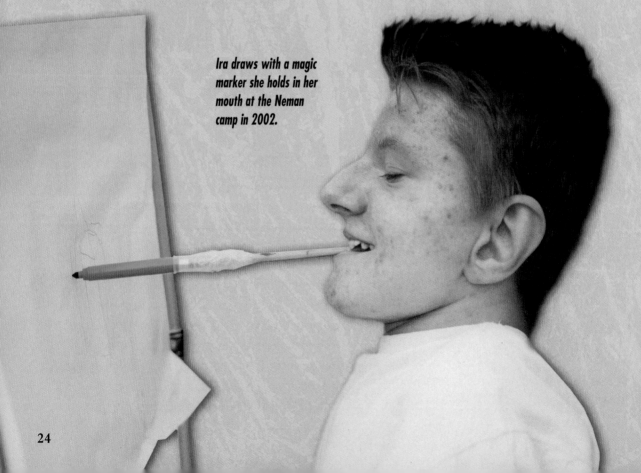

Ira draws with a magic marker she holds in her mouth at the Neman camp in 2002.

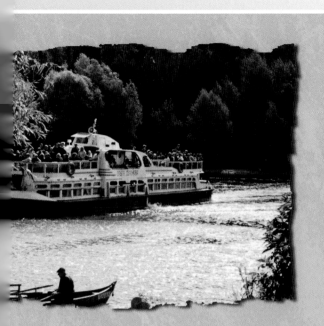

At the Neman camp, the children are taken for walks in the woods, rides down the river on a boat, and on outings to the zoo or the park.

HELPING CHERNOBYL'S CHILDREN

People who volunteer at the vacation camp play a vital role in giving the children a wonderful three weeks.

• Most volunteers at the camp are young people, and they include many medical and physical-therapy students. Some volunteers have previously worked with children or with people with special needs as teachers, play workers, or physical therapists.

• Other volunteers are just enthusiastic, caring people eager to make a difference to the lives of so many children.

• The vacations are sometimes life changing for the volunteers. Many have been inspired to change their college major or their job so that they can work with children with special needs in the future.

• Having so many volunteers and caregivers at the camp allows children with severe physical disabilities, like Ira, and children with profound learning difficulties to enjoy one-to-one support in a way that would never be possible at a home like Zhuravichi.

HELEN WALKER SAYS:

"I was sixteen the first time I volunteered at the holiday camp. The kids were amazing and I loved every minute of it. But when we had to say goodbye it was awful because we didn't know what life we were sending them back to. Was it cruel to give them all that love and then say, 'Goodbye, see you in a year'? I wasn't sure, until I visited them in their orphanage a few months later. All any of the children could say to me was, 'When are we going to the holiday camp again? Am I going? Are you going? Is she going?' It made me realize just how much of a difference the holidays make to the children's lives. I've now volunteered every summer for the past six years."

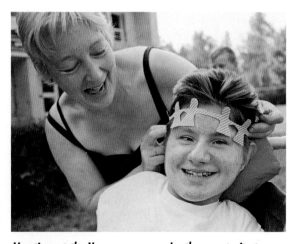

Vacations at the Neman camp gave Ira the opportunity to meet lots of new people.

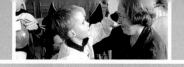

Living After Chernobyl

LINDA WALKER SAYS:

"Ira's first holiday away from Zhuravichi opened her eyes to what she might be capable of if she was given the opportunity. When she returned to Zhuravichi, she was desperate to be able to read and to have a chance to know more about the world outside the orphanage. In 2003, we arranged with Raisa, the director of Zhuravichi, for some of the most disabled children to be taught by one of the Zhuravichi teachers, Ludmilla Markovna. That spring, Ira found herself in a classroom for the first time in her life, and later that year, we were able to arrange for her to go to live at the Rechitsa Boarding School, near to the city of Gomel."

IRA SAYS:

"After I came back from my first vacation, it seemed very quiet in my room at Zhuravichi.

My head was so full of stories about my new friends and the things I had done. I was bursting to talk about the vacation.

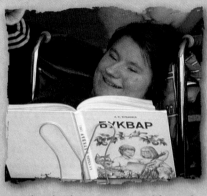

Ira loved to have someone read fairy tales to her, but she wanted to be able to read them on her own.

I liked to sit in the corridor so I could sometimes chat to children from other parts of the building because the children in my group could not really talk. Sometimes Natalia Nicolaevna came to talk to me. Natalia was my favorite caregiver but then she became deputy director.

I was very happy when I started to have lessons with Ludmilla Markovna. She read me stories and taught me to count, and I learned to read new words every day.

One day, Natalia came to tell me I was going to leave Zhuravichi and go to live at Rechitsa Boarding School. I was upset to think of leaving Natalia and Ludmilla, but Vova was going, too, and Peter and Ghenya and Alina. And I would meet some of my friends from the holiday again.

Ludmilla Markovna works with some of her pupils at Zhuravichi.

It was exciting and frightening at the same time. I would miss everyone at Zhuravichi, but I wanted to go to study."

LUDMILLA MARKOVNA SAYS:

"I soon found that it was a pleasure to teach Ira. She had a hunger for information and loved to listen to stories about people and relationships. When we looked at pictures, she wanted to know everything about them. Ira liked to play with words and syllables. Lots of children find it hard to learn all the different endings on Russian words, and foreigners hate it! But Ira just loves the sound of words.

It was rewarding to teach Ira. It was not like running water through a sieve, the work brought good fruit, and her face would shine with happiness when she thanked me for teaching her."

EDUCATION IN BELARUS

In Belarus, most children start school at six years old. In many schools, especially in country villages, the buildings are not big enough to accommodate all the pupils at once. Half the children start school early, at 8:00 A.M., and finish in the early afternoon. Then, a second shift starts and goes on into the evening. Children in Belarus are expected to take school very seriously. They study hard, rarely misbehave in school, and have lots of homework. Many schools in contaminated areas stayed open after the Chernobyl accident, but the students were not allowed to play outside if a school's playground was radioactive.

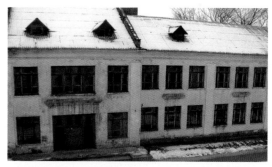

This school in a contaminated part of Belarus was abandoned after the local population was evacuated.

SPECIAL-NEEDS EDUCATION

In the past, education for Belarussian children with special needs was not of very high quality. Children were assessed at five years old and could be labeled as having "oligophrenia," or "few brains." Children with very severe disabilities were often pronounced unteachable. Those said to have oligophrenia were not allowed to go to ordinary schools. As adults, they would have difficulty getting jobs because employers were reluctant to hire people with their "problem." Some of the children given this label did not have learning problems but just had a bad start in life because of parents who were alcoholic or uncaring. In spite of this, it was very rare for children to be reassessed and moved to mainstream schools. There is now a law in Belarus that says that all children must be taught.

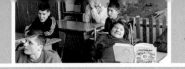

IRA SAYS:

"When I went to camp for the second time [in the summer of 2003], I knew I would soon be moving to Rechitsa School. I spent as much time as I could with girls from the school and made some friends. [Children from the Rechitsa Boarding School also go to the Neman holiday camp.] Just a week after we got back to Zhuravichi, we left for Rechitsa. The five of us [Ira, Vova, Peter, Ghenya, and Alina] were dressed in our best clothes, we said goodbye to our friends and then we were put into the van for the journey to the school. I cried when I said goodbye to Natalia Nicolaevna, and she cried, too. The journey to Rechitsa took two hours, and I felt sad all the way.

When we arrived, we were quickly put into the isolation room. A doctor told us it was in case we had any illnesses which we might give to the other children. I wanted to see the girls I knew from the vacation and to have my first lesson, but we had to stay in this room for a week. I wondered if it would have been better to stay at Zhuravichi.

One morning, we were all taken from the isolation room to the school hall. This is a very big room, and all the children in the school were there. The caregivers gave me a wheelchair, and I watched some of the children singing. Then I was taken to a classroom where I met my teacher. There were about eight other children in the class, but none of them could speak. I felt very shy, and when the teacher asked me questions, I just said, 'yes' or 'no' or 'OK.'"

ELENA VALERIEVNA SAYS:

"I was Ira's first teacher when she came to Rechitsa. It took two or three weeks before Ira would really talk to us. Eventually, she relaxed and started to answer

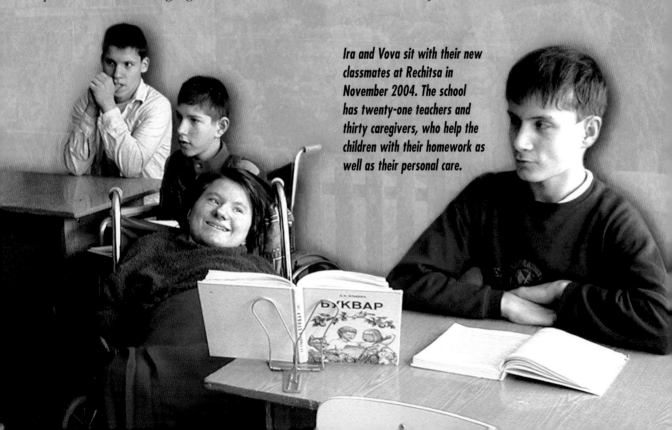

Ira and Vova sit with their new classmates at Rechitsa in November 2004. The school has twenty-one teachers and thirty caregivers, who help the children with their homework as well as their personal care.

our questions about how she felt and what she wanted. It seemed she spent most of the time in bed at Zhuravichi. She told me she was worried that she was going to stay in the quarantine bed at Rechitsa! Now Ira has a nice bed, with a special, thick mattress, in a room she shares with five other girls. We gave her a bedside table and put a framed picture of her on the wall. She was so pleased. Then she started to 'defrost.'

Recently, Ira was moved to a new class where all the children can speak. At the moment, she is below the level of the other children in her new class, so she is like a sponge, absorbing everything!"

THE RECHITSA BOARDING SCHOOL

Many pupils at the Rechitsa Boarding School are taught the mainstream national curriculum. The children with learning difficulties follow an adapted special-needs program. All the children are encouraged to work as hard as they can. Sports, gymnastics, drama, art, and music are also important at Rechitsa, and the children's talents in all these areas are recognized and developed.

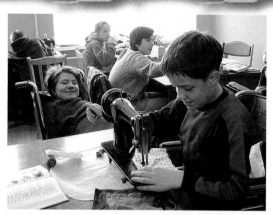

Ira sits in on a sewing class at the Rechitsa school.

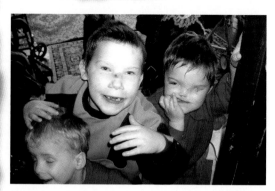

The children at Rechitsa range in age from five to eighteen.

SOCIAL ORPHANS

A total of 106 children attend school at Rechitsa. Half of them never see their parents. These children are known as "social orphans." Some of them, such as Ira, were abandoned by their parents because of the child's disabilities. Other children were taken away from parents who have severe alcohol problems. Living with poverty and anxiety about health problems, disabilities, and what the future will hold has led to widespread alcoholism in the regions affected by the Chernobyl disaster. Vodka is inexpensive in this part of the world, and alcohol abuse was initially made worse by official advice that "Vodka helps to protect you from radiation."

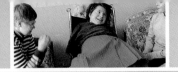

CHAPTER FOUR: Ira's Life Today

Millions of people from Belarus, Ukraine, and parts of Russia live with the consequences of the Chernobyl disaster every day of their lives. At places such as Zhuravichi and Rechitsa, however, the accident and its effects are very rarely discussed. The staff feel the children have enough to worry about as they cope with their disabilities and come to terms with the difficult future that is ahead of them.

IRA SAYS:

"I still can't believe there is really going to be a book about me. My friends are all quite excited, and I hope they will all be in the book, too. I like looking at books about other children and hearing their stories. And, now, children will be able to read about me. I never imagined such a thing could be possible!

In this picture from November 2004, Ira wears colorful clothes. Some of the Rechitsa children's clothes are bought by the school. Overseas charities also send aid to schools and orphanages in Belarus, including lots of bright, colorful clothes.

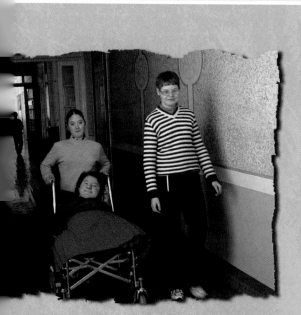

Ira's friend Luba (left) pushes Ira in her wheelchair, as another friend, Tanya, walks beside her. Unlike many wheelchair users, Ira cannot use her arms to move her chair around. She relies on her friends and caregivers to push her everywhere.

I like to see myself in photographs. When we chose a picture for the wall in my room, my friends said they liked the ones with me smiling best. They were right, so now I always try to smile when someone takes my picture.

I always like to dress up in pretty clothes— have a bow put in my hair, wear something fluffy. I like skirts, and my favorite color is red. I wore my red skirt for a lot of the photos for this book. I like to wear perfume, and sometimes at the holiday camp the volunteers put make-up on me and colors on my nails. It made me feel very grown-up.

At Rechitsa, my friends Luba and Tanya help me to look pretty. It is exciting when visitors come. We all get dressed up and look as neat as we can."

BELARUS TODAY: HEALTH

Government resources in Belarus are still overstretched when it comes to caring for orphans and disabled children.

• Belarussian hospitals lack resources, from diapers and sterile needles to expensive medicines and incubators for maternity wards.

• In the Gomel region, births of disabled children have increased by 80 percent, even though women are encouraged to terminate pregnancies if any damage to the fetus is suspected.

• The World Health Organization (WHO) predicts that one-third of all Gomel region inhabitants who were four years old or younger at the time of the Chernobyl accident will develop thyroid cancer. The WHO expects this to equal fifty thousand cases in this one area of Belarus alone. Some radiation experts think that prediction is low. They estimate there will be one hundred thousand cases.

• A UNICEF analysis of Belarussian health statistics showed that between 1990 and 1994, disorders of the nervous system in children increased by 43 percent, cardiovascular diseases by 43 percent, gastrointestinal diseases by 28 percent, disorders of bone, muscle, and connective tissue by 62 percent, and diabetes by 28 percent.

• Cases of breast cancer in the Gomel region have doubled.

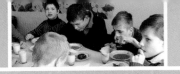

"I enjoy summertime best, when it is warm and we can spend lots of time outside. My friends push me around, or we sit under a tree and talk. You don't have to wear lots of clothes in the summer, and I am much more comfortable. It is too cold to be outside in the winter, and my wheelchair is too hard to push in the snow.

I like animals. We have a cat named Malysh and a dog, Sharik, in our school yard, and I like to feed them with pieces of my bread. We also have fish in the aquarium, which I enjoy watching, and a hamster.

There are lots of activities at Rechitsa. I like pop music, especially fast music, and I love to go to dances. We have lots of dances at the holiday camp and also here in school. Last Sunday, I was reading a book with Galina, my caregiver. I was enjoying the book, but when they put the music on in the hall, and Galina asked if I wanted to keep reading or go to the dance, it wasn't hard to decide. I went straight to the dance! I try to move to the music, but I can't move much on my own, so I like it when someone swings my wheelchair in time to the music. It is fun when the grown-ups dance.

I like watching TV. We get to watch television every afternoon or evening, and I love to see concerts and musical films. My favorite film is called Clone—it is about friends. I like to listen to people reading fairy tales, too.

I like any food, but my favorites are fried meat and sausage and bread and butter. My favorite lunch is draniki. It is made from grated potatoes and meat. I also like fruit and chocolates and other sweets. We usually get some sweets over the weekend. The food is nice here—tastier than it was at Zhuravichi.

One of the caregivers at Rechitsa feeds Ira because Ira cannot use her hands at all.

My favorite subjects in school are reading and reciting poems. I like to learn poems by heart, and I also enjoy studying Russian, but I find Belarussian really hard. Music lessons are fun, and I quite like math, but reading is definitely my favorite subject.

I am learning about religion. We have a priest who comes into school, and I like to listen to him. Some of the children talk about God a lot. But I just listen. I don't think God can change my life.

I like it here. I am happy. But I still miss Natalia Nicolaevna and Ludmilla Markovna."

A TYPICAL DAY AT RECHITSA

The children wake up at 7:30 A.M., get washed and dressed, and have breakfast in the canteen at about 8:30 A.M. Lessons take place between 9:00 A.M. and 1:30 P.M. At the end of the morning, the children have lunch in the canteen. In the afternoon, it is homework time. Ira's friend, Luba, has three or four hours of homework to do every day. Ira does not have that much work to do, but she practices reciting poems, and a caregiver helps her with her reading. In the evening, after a meal at 7:00 P.M., the children sit with friends and chat, listen to music, or watch films on TV until they are ready for bed.

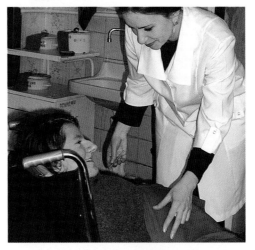

Doctors are a permanent part of the staff at Rechitsa. Ira has regular massage and heat therapy to ease her back pains.

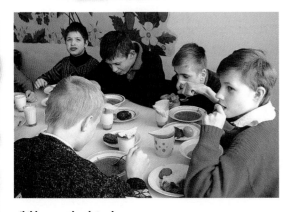

Children eat lunch in the canteen.

MEALTIMES AT RECHITSA

At Rechitsa, the children eat their meals in the canteen. A typical breakfast is baked cottage cheese with potatoes and some salad. The children usually have soup at lunchtime, followed by a dinner of pasta or potatoes with pork or chicken and locally grown vegetables. Sometimes, in the summer, fruit is available, but, in winter, fruit is a rare treat.

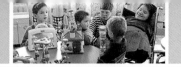

IRA SAYS:

"The children here at Rechitsa are very nice and kind. They treat me well. They take me where I ask them to, they put the television on for me, and they get the caregiver to come if I need her.

I have lots of friends. When I was younger, I liked to play school with my special friend, Vova. I was always the teacher. Sometimes we learned poems together. I would say one line, then Vova would say the next. We still spend a lot of time together, as Vova is at the same school as me.

Here at Rechitsa, my best friends are the girls I share my room with, Luba and Tanya. I like to sit in the bedroom with Luba and Tanya and just chat. We talk about other friends, about what we have done in class, and about the teachers."

VOVA SAYS:

"When we were little, I used to push Ira about. I also helped to feed her sometimes. If I did anything wrong, like feeding her too fast, she used to shout at me. It upset me because I was only trying to be helpful. I think Ludmilla Markovna talked to Ira about it, and then she became more patient. After that, we used to play games where Ira was the caregiver or teacher, and she used to order me about then, too, but that was just for fun!"

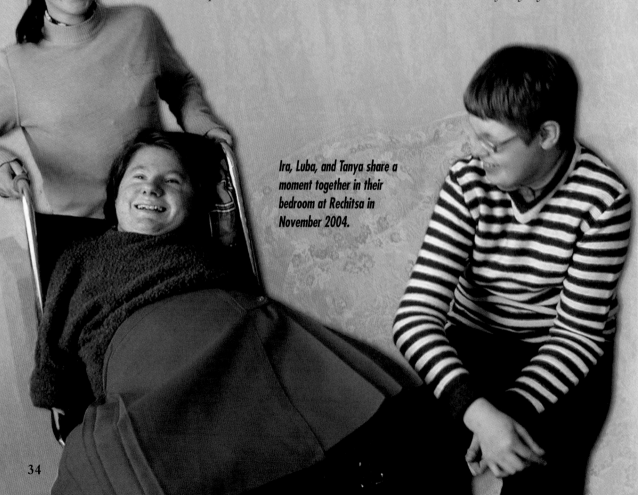

Ira, Luba, and Tanya share a moment together in their bedroom at Rechitsa in November 2004.

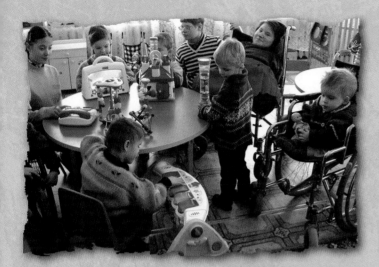

Luba, Tanya, and Ira spend time with some of Rechitsa's younger children in the school's playroom.

ABOUT IRA

During the preparation for this book, Liena Fedarchuk, who works with CCP (UK) in Gomel, spoke to many people who have known Ira over the years. Everyone had something to say about Ira that they wanted included in the book.

"Ira is very talkative, but she never says anything bad about people. She never interrupts and would not shout. She is tactful, to put it in one word." (Ludmilla Markovna)

"In general, if Ira does not like something, she would rather keep silent about it than say anything negative. Though Ira has a disability, she is kind toward other people and always smiles. I think she views the world around her very positively and is always very appreciative. We went for a walk outdoors recently, and I treated her to an apple. It was enough to make her happy." (Elena Valerievna, Ira's teacher at Rechitsa Boarding School)

"Ira has a very strong character and is a very purposeful person. She wants to live, and she lives in the present." (Deputy Head, Rechitsa Boarding School)

"Ira can be happy about a single day. If there is something good, then she is happy. If not, she might not even think about it tomorrow. Ira has a thirst for life and takes life as it is today." (Galina, Ira's caregiver at Rechitsa Boarding School)

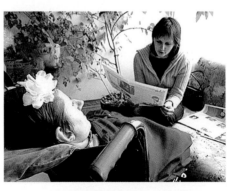

Liena Fedarchuk reads Ira the first draft of this book, translating the English text into Russian.

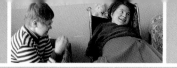

IRA SAYS:

"Some days I think about my mother. I understand why she could not look after me, but I wish I could see her. I sometimes see a TV program called Where Are They Now? It helps people to find each other. I was hoping that my mother could be found through the program, but my teacher said no one knows an address for her, so it is too difficult.

Some of the children here [at Rechitsa] have mothers who come to visit them, and some have fathers, too. I am happy for them when their mothers come to visit, and I like to talk to their parents, but it makes me feel empty.

I hope my mother is still alive. Maybe one day I will meet her."

LUDMILLA MARKOVNA SAYS:

"All our children [at Zhuravichi] who are able to speak and understand what is happening around them are desperate to talk about their family. Often they ask, 'Why is my mother not coming back for me? What does she do? What is her job?'

Ira lies in her bed at the Rechitsa Boarding School in November 2004.

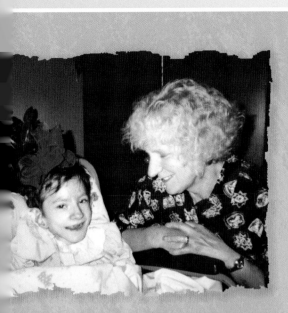

In this picture from 1999, Ira is dressed up for visitors. The staff at Zhuravichi became Ira's family, and while she was there, Ira liked to talk with them about their husbands and children.

So we use imagination to talk to the children about their families.

Ira has never had any fantasies about her mother. She is a more rational girl.

A few years ago, I was in the eye hospital and met a blind woman from the next ward who was originally from Tihinichi village, near Rogachev. Ira's mother was supposed to have come from that village.

The woman told me about her severely disabled daughter who died. So, being a Sherlock Holmes in my heart, I thought for a while that she could have been Ira's mother. But, then, it appeared that the lady's name was Pirozhkova, while Ira's was Rozhkova."

BELARUS TODAY: THE SOCIAL AND ECONOMIC COSTS

It is projected that the cost to Belarus for the first thirty years after the accident (1986–2015) will be U.S. $235 billion. This is the equivalent of thirty-two annual budgets for the country. The government of Belarus had to pay for cleaning up the contaminated area after the disaster. It also lost revenues from industries that had to shut down as a result of the disaster.

• In the contaminated areas of Belarus, fifty-four large agricultural and forestry enterprises have had to close, together with nine industrial enterprises and twenty-two raw-material mines.

• Most of the people who have left (and are still leaving) the affected areas are young families. In these areas, there is now a shortage of teachers and doctors. Companies and farms in the affected areas are also closing because of a lack of skilled workers.

• In spite of financial help from the government, agriculture is no longer profitable for many farmers in the contaminated regions. Even produce that has been strictly monitored and certified as safe is difficult to sell.

• In 1986, the population of Gomel was increasing by 8 percent a year. Today, the birth rate in the region is dropping and mortality has increased. In 2000, the population in the region shrank by 5.1 percent.

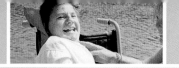

CHAPTER FIVE: Looking to the Future

No one knows how many children have been born severely disabled as a result of the Chernobyl accident. All we can say for sure is that, even though fewer children are being born in regions such as Gomel, the number of children born with disabilities has significantly increased. Ira is now sixteen years old. She knows that her life will never be easy and that she will always need people to look after her.

LINDA WALKER SAYS:

"One of Ira's caregivers at Rechitsa told us this story about a discussion that was had one day in class. Zhenya, one of the boys at Rechitsa, was about to have a throat operation, so we talked with the children about it. Ira asked what the operation was for. So I told her there is a hope that Zhenya can start talking, he might be better after the operation. Ira asked, 'Is there no operation that can help me?' I told Ira, 'I think not, but you can be happy that even though you cannot walk and write, you are able to talk. Zhenya walks and writes but is not able to talk. In a way, it is simpler for you as you can say what you would like to happen, while Zhenya has to use gestures.'

Ira was very quiet for about fifteen minutes. Then she said, 'You know, you're right.' I could not understand what she was talking about, so I went and sat near her. Ira said, 'Nothing, no operation can help me, but I feel good. I am happy that I can speak.'

Ira assessed her real abilities. She understands that nothing can help her, so she does not upset

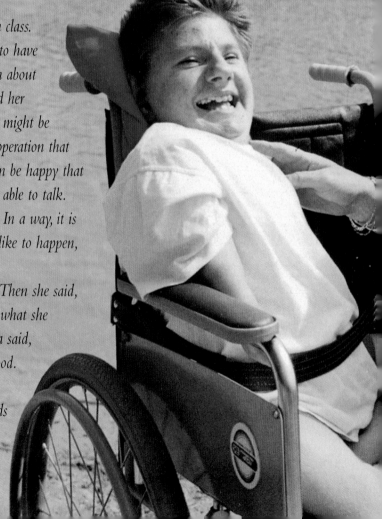

FAMILY HOME 2000

When young, disabled people leave orphanages, they usually move into adult boarding institutions where there is often very little for the residents to do. In 2000, CCP (UK) set up a small home in which four young adults with physical disabilities (Liena, Greesha, Sasha, and Sveta) could live in a family environment. They have learned to cook and take care of themselves, and they are all learning trades that will help them to become more independent in the future.

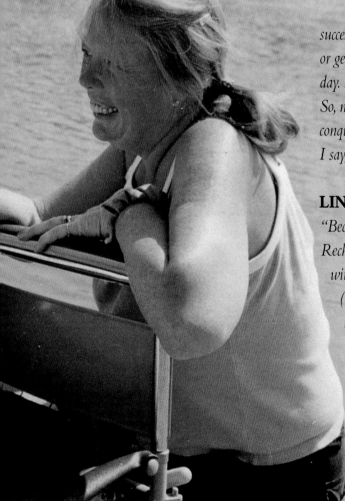

herself about it. She does not feel that God took any abilities off her. I think Ira believes that we are all different. She is not disabled, not defective, but individual. She is like she is."

IRA SAYS:

"I don't really think about what will happen in the future. I know I will leave Rechitsa and go to another home, but I don't know where. Sometimes I think about being at Zhuravichi and being in a cot where none of the children around me could speak. I feel very lucky to be here at Rechitsa.

I am happiest when I do something, and it is successful. But if I fail in something, I do not panic or get upset. I try to believe tomorrow will be a better day. For a while I would say, 'I cannot do that today.' So, my teacher at Rechitsa said to me, 'We need to conquer the cannot.' Now, when there is a difficulty, I say, 'Let's conquer the cannot!'"

LINDA WALKER SAYS:

"Because Ira made such a late start to her studies, Rechitsa Boarding School is happy to let her stay with them until she is twenty. After that, CCP (UK) is hoping that it will be possible for Ira to move into their "Family Home 2000," in Klimovka, just outside Gomel."

Ira talks with Glenda Tracey, a volunteer, during her first vacation at the Neman holiday camp in 2002.

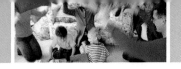

LIVING WITH THE RADIATION MONSTER

In 2006, it will be twenty years since the Chernobyl accident, but time has not been a healer for the people of the Chernobyl region. Many children living in the affected areas in Belarus, Ukraine, and Russia think a great deal about Chernobyl and worry about the effect it will have on their future lives. Tamara was twelve years old and lived in a village called Uvaravichi, near to the city of Gomel, when she traveled to northern England for a vacation. She wrote a card to thank her host family for the visit saying, "It seems to me that Chernobyl is like a great big monster trying to destroy us, and the English families are our fairy godmothers helping to protect us from the radiation monster."

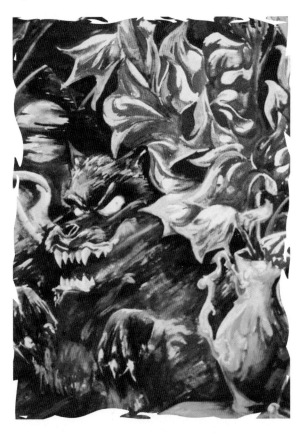

This painting was created by teenagers in Belarus. The monster represents Chernobyl eating up the beautiful world.

TOMORROW'S CHERNOBYL CHILDREN

Today, doctors in the most contaminated parts of Belarus report that only 10 percent of children born in these areas are completely healthy. Teenagers living in these areas are very frightened about what will happen when they get married and have children of their own. Many young people seek the opportunity to go and live abroad, where they hope they can improve their health and where their children will have a better chance of being born healthy in the future. Young men and women who were little children at the time of the accident are now becoming parents. Many young women are experiencing problems during pregnancy or labor, and there has been an increase in the number of children born with genetic defects.

NO END IN SIGHT

Many children still live in tiny rural villages, sometimes just a few miles from the Chernobyl plant. In the early years after the accident, people were very anxious about the effects of radiation, especially on their children, and they tried hard to find uncontaminated food to eat. It is hard, however, for parents and caregivers to be vigilant for many years about a hazard they cannot see, taste, or smell. Many poor families have started to collect mushrooms in the forests again and hunt wild animals to supplement their diets. These foods are very high in cesium-137, and this radioactive substance is absorbed into children's bodies. Eating contaminated food day after day causes the amount of radiation in the body to grow. Children living in these conditions may not be ill yet, but their future is bleak if they continue to live in such a dangerous environment.

HELPING THE CHERNOBYL CHILDREN

Charities from all over the world continue to help children in the affected regions. They deliver humanitarian aid; bring children out of Belarus,

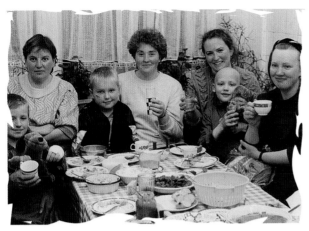

Mothers and children share a meal at a hostel run by the Minsk cancer charity, Children in Trouble. Families stay at the hostel while children are undergoing cancer treatment in Minsk.

Ukraine, and Russia for recuperative vacations; and help to support orphanages or hospitals, often by sending out teams of volunteers to work on building projects. Many of the children who enjoy respite vacations are in remission from leukemia or cancer. Vacations abroad are especially important for these children—particularly those in their teens, many of whom become sick for a second or third time and have a high death rate. A happy, healthy summer vacation may give them a better chance of survival.

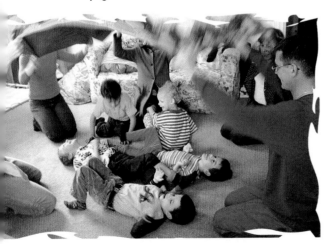

These young disabled children live in the small "family" home set up by CCP (UK) in Rogachev, Belarus. Papa Sergei (right) has become the children's legal guardian. The children are cared for by caregivers known as "aunties."

CHERNOBYL CHILDREN'S PROJECT (UK)

The charity Chernobyl Children's Project (UK) helps children in Belarus. It is one of the many organizations dedicated to improving the lives of children affected by the Chernobyl disaster. The organization works closely with homes for children with disabilities such as the Abandoned Babies' Home, Zhuravichi Children's Home, and Rechitsa Boarding School.

• CCP (UK) aid convoys deliver medical aid, school equipment, disability aids, toys, toiletries, diapers, and bedding.

• CCP (UK) has established a small "family" home in which young disabled adults can gain some independence. It has also set up a home for disabled children, in which a small number of children live with "aunties" (caregivers) in a setting that is like a normal family.

• CCP (UK) funds children's hospice care and organizes training for hospice nurses. It has also run a training program to help orphanage staff members place children into foster care with local families.

• In 2004, CCP (UK) opened a center in Gomel where severely disabled children who are normally cared for by their families can stay while their families take a break from the hard work of caring for their children.

• Many of these projects have been undertaken in close cooperation with the local authorities in the Gomel region, who are enthusiastic about creating a better future for children with special needs.

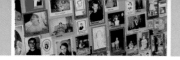

CHAPTER SIX: Those Who Help

The Chernobyl disaster has directly or indirectly affected the lives of nine million people in Belarus, Ukraine, and Russia. At least three million of those people are children. Following the Chernobyl accident, many feared there could be another disaster as large as Chernobyl.

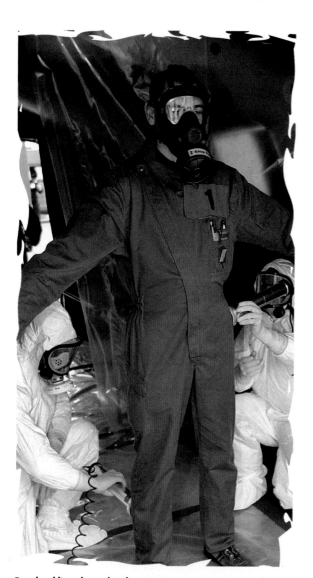

French soldiers dressed in decontamination suits measure radioactivity levels during a drill in which a nuclear accident was simulated.

THE ULTIMATE ENERGY SOURCE?

In the 1950s and 1960s, the world looked to nuclear power as a cheap, renewable source of energy. A little bit more than 2 pounds (1 kilogram) of uranium could power a whole city, without producing any of the pollution associated with burning fossil fuels. As the nuclear-power industry grew, however, so did concerns about its safety. Scientists learned that, even in small doses, radiation can cause cancer and the disposal of fuel rods, which stay radioactive for thousands of years, became an increasing cause of worry. In the aftermath of the Chernobyl disaster, huge public and political pressure and the costs of new design and safety rules limited the expansion of the nuclear power industry.

THE FUTURE OF NUCLEAR POWER

Today, many people in large, industrialized countries, such as the United States, see renewed investment in nuclear power as the only way forward in a world that needs energy sources that do not produce greenhouse gases. Many scientists, however, point out that the nuclear fuel cycle does, in fact, produce carbon dioxide.

In Belarus, a desperately poor country that has to import nearly all of its energy, there are calls for the country to build its own new, modern nuclear power stations. Russia currently has thirty nuclear

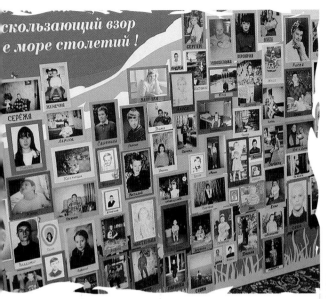

The "Memory Room" at a children's hospice in Minsk, Belarus.

eactors in operation and is planning eight new ones.

Ukraine remains committed to nuclear power, relying on nuclear energy for 45 percent of its electricity needs. Thirteen nuclear power stations currently operate, with two new plants soon to be completed—in spite of warnings from overseas nuclear experts that defects could affect the safety of the new plants.

THE "SARCOPHAGUS"

At the Chernobyl power station, reactor Unit 4 remains enclosed in its reinforced, concrete "sarcophagus." Hastily built and potentially unstable, the sarcophagus was designed to last only twenty to thirty years. In 2003, the Russian Atomic Energy minister, Alexander Rumyantsev, reported that the structure could collapse at any time. An internationally funded project to build a new 328-foot (100-meter) high, 22,040-pound (20,000-metric ton) steel shelter is now underway. The new shelter should be completed by 2008 and will keep the

Unit 4 reactor contained for at least one hundred years. During that time, an even longer lasting solution will have to be found.

THE HEALTH IMPACTS

The full impact of the Chernobyl accident on the health of the people living in the affected regions is impossible to quantify. Even though doctors know that exposure to radiation can cause cancer, genetic mutations, and many other medical problems, there is no way to prove for sure whether a particular health problem was caused by radiation or by some other cause.

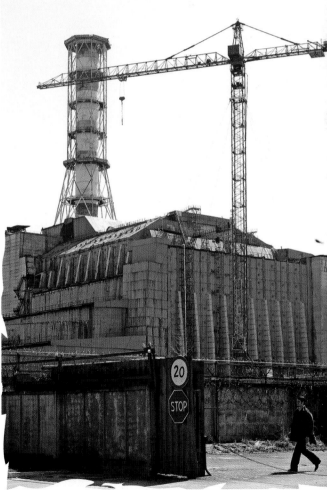

This concrete sarcophagus was built in 1986 to hold Chernobyl power station's Unit 4 nuclear reactor.

43

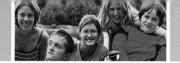

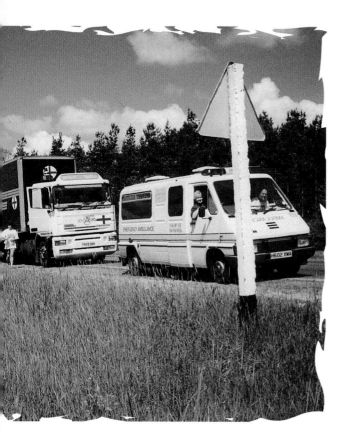

A CCP (UK) aid convoy drives across Europe to deliver humanitarian aid to Belarus.

The number of casualties, therefore, remains controversial. Experts now agree, however, that the Chernobyl disaster caused many cancers and, in particular, thyroid cancers. The full medical impact of Chernobyl will not be known until at least 2016.

INTERNATIONAL AID'

Because of the Soviet government's initial secrecy surrounding the accident, it was 1989 before the full damage done by the disaster became clear to the international community. In 1990, the United Nations (UN) set up an Inter-Agency Task Force on Chernobyl. It was set up to raise funds and manage projects that would help to deal with the harm done by the Chernobyl accident in the affected regions. Since 2001, aid projects have focused on medical programs for the people most affected (women, children, and liquidators) and projects that "help people to help themselves" through economic aid and practical assistance in dealing with radioactive contamination. Many of the current health-care projects emphasize early diagnosis and treatment of thyroid cancer and other cancers in children. These projects are often jointly funded by governments and charities. According to the UN, tens of billions of dollars are still needed to help the millions of people living in contaminated areas.

HELP FROM CHARITIES

Around the world, many charities and nonprofit social service agencies are raising money and working directly with the people of Belarus, Ukraine, and Russia. To date, these organizations have arranged for more than half a million children to travel abroad for respite vacations. In addition, thirty-eight cities and communities across Europe are "sisters" with places in the Chernobyl region. These cities work with their Chernobyl sisters to help improve the lives of people living with the ongoing effects of the disaster.

THE CHERNOBYL REGION

Today, almost four hundred thousand people from the areas affected by the Chernobyl disaster are considered environmental refugees, or people who have had to leave their homes as a result of an environmental disaster. More than two thousand towns and villages have been abandoned, bulldozed, or buried. In spite of laws against it, at least eight hundred people, most of whom are elderly, have returned to live in villages inside the exclusion zone. They choose to live with the dangers of radiation rather than live in unfamiliar cities. Scientists predict it will not be safe to live in the exclusion zone until the year 2300. Areas in the Chernobyl region contaminated with plutonium will be uninhabitable forever.

LIVING WITH CHERNOBYL

In the future, it is vital that governments around the world maintain a commitment to the residents of the towns and villages around Chernobyl. It is essential that greater research into the health effects of the accident take place and that every effort is made to ensure that the Chernobyl Unit 4 reactor is made completely safe for the future.

Today, more than 430 nuclear power stations are currently in operation worldwide, with more under construction. At the time of the Chernobyl accident, Soviet government officials said that the odds of a meltdown at the Chernobyl plant were one in ten thousand.

In a 2001 statement, five scientists from the Ukraine Ministry of Health summed up the disaster in the following 2001 statement: "The Chernobyl radiation accident is undoubtedly the greatest environmental catastrophe in the history of mankind." The world must never forget the children of Chernobyl, the generations yet to come, and the terrible events of Saturday, April 26, 1986.

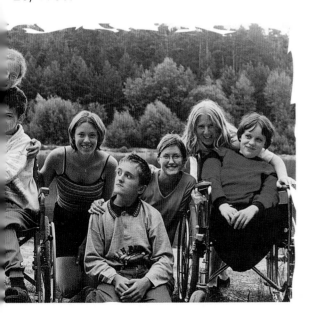

Belarussian teenagers and volunteers at the Neman vacation camp pose for a picture together in 2000.

HOW YOU CAN HELP

1. ORGANIZE A COLLECTION OF TOYS

Lego and other educational toys are always desperately needed by orphanages and hospitals.

2. ORGANIZE A FUNDRAISER

Funds are desperately needed to continue helping children like Ira:
• About $40 will transport ten humanitarian-aid boxes to Belarus on one of CCP (UK)'s trucks.
• About $110 will pay one month's salary for one caregiver at CCP (UK)'s new respite care home.
• Consider holding a fundraiser at your school to help pay for a child's summer vacation. About $365 will pay for a child's airfare from Belarus to Britain for a vacation that will boost the child's immune system.

3. BE INFORMED ABOUT THE ISSUES AND RAISE AWARENESS

Sign up on the Web site of one of the groups that works to help victims of the Chernobyl disaster to receive regular newsletters, and pass along the information you receive to as many people as possible.

4. SEND A PICTURE TO IRA

Send a picture of yourself, your family, and your friends to Ira so she and her friends will know that you have read this book. Pictures can be sent to CCP (UK).

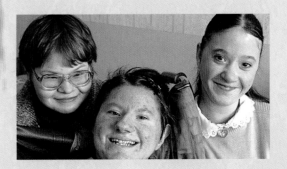

Glossary

AUTISM A developmental disorder that can be characterized by impairment of the ability to form social relationships, impairment of ability to communicate with others, or the presence of particular behavioral patterns.

CANCER A disease in which cells reproduce in an uncontrolled manner and interfere with the normal function of the body's systems.

CEREBRAL PALSY A disability characterized by problems with speech and muscular coordination that is caused by damage to the brain before, during, or soon after birth.

CESIUM-137 A radioactive isotope with a half-life of thirty years.

CORE The tough, steel container at the heart of a nuclear reactor containing uranium fuel rods in which nuclear fission takes place.

DNA The molecule that serves as the basis for heredity.

DOWN SYNDROME A congenital condition marked by moderate to severe mental retardation and a distinctive physical appearance that includes slanting eyes and a broad, short skull.

FALLOUT The often radioactive particles that descend through the atmosphere as a result of a nuclear explosion.

FUEL ROD A rod containing uranium used as the fuel in a nuclear reactor; used fuel rods remain dangerously radioactive.

HALF-LIFE The time taken for the radioactivity of an isotope to fall to half its value.

HOT SPOT A place of greater than usual interest or activity; in the areas affected by Chernobyl, a place with higher than usual radioactivity.

IODINE-131 A radioactive isotope with a half-life of eight days.

ISOTOPE A form of an element that has most of the characteristics of the pure element but differs in its properties and its radioactivity.

LEUKEMIA A form of cancer affecting the blood producing cells in bone marrow; radioactive strontium-90 collects in bones and is thought to cause leukemia.

MAGNITUDE Large size or great extent.

MELTDOWN An accident in which the core of a nuclear reactor melts.

NUCLEAR FISSION The energy-producing process by which atomic nuclei are split apart.

PLUTONIUM A radioactive element that is used in nuclear reactors; some plutonium isotopes have half-lives of up to twenty-four thousand years.

RADIOACTIVE Emitting radiation.

RADIOACTIVITY The capability of an atom of giving off energetic particles, such as electrons, as the atom's nucleus disintegrates; the energy given off is called radiation.

RADIONULCIDE A radioactive atom characterized by the contents of its nucleus in terms of number of protons, neutrons, and energy content.

REACTOR An installation at a nuclear power plant in which the nuclear fission reaction takes place.

SARCOPHAGUS A stone coffin; used to describe the mostly concrete structure that has been built to contain the radioactive remains of Chernobyl Unit 4.

SOVIET UNION A former federation of fifteen communist countries occupying the northern half of Asia and part of Eastern Europe; also known as the Union of Soviet Socialist Republics (USSR).

SPINA BIFIDA A hereditary disorder of the backbone.

STRONTIUM-90 A radioactive isotope that has a half-life of thirty years.

TURBINE A machine that spins and produces electricity.

UNICEF The United Nations Children's Fund; an agency of the UN established to help governments improve the health, lives, and education of the world's children.

UNITED NATIONS (UN) An international organization of countries set up in 1945 to promote international peace, security, and cooperation.

URANIUM A radioactive element; uranium isotopes are used as fuel in nuclear reactors and create, as a byproduct, plutonium, which can be used in nuclear power and in atomic weapons.

VICINITY Surrounding area or neighborhood.

Further Information

CHABAD'S CHILDREN OF CHERNOBYL

This charity evacuates children from the contaminated areas of Belarus and Ukraine and sends them to Israel for medical care, nutrition, and education. More than two thousand children have received medical attention through the efforts of this organization.
www.ccoc.net

CHERNOBYL CHILDREN'S PROJECT (UK)

Chernobyl Children's Project (UK) provides vacations for hundreds of children suffering from cancer and leukemia as a result of the Chernobyl disaster. The project also delivers medical supplies and basic necessities to Belarus.
www.chernobyl-children.org.uk

CHERNOBYL CHILDREN'S PROJECT INTERNATIONAL

A nonprofit organization that provides aid to the millions of children made sick by the Chernobyl disaster and works with the UN to increase awareness of Chernobyl's impact on Belarussians.
www.ccp-intl.org

CHILDREN OF CHORNOBYL RELIEF AND DEVELOPMENT FUND

The goal of this organization is to provide state-of-the-art medical aid to children suffering from cancer, heart disease, birth defects, and other diseases as a result of the Chernobyl disaster. A map on its Web site shows the hospitals in the Ukraine being helped by this charity's efforts.
www.childrenofchornobyl.org

INTERNATIONAL CHERNOBYL RESEARCH INFORMATION NETWORK (ICRIN)

This Web site shows the long-term consequences of the 1986 reactor explosion in Chernobyl and provides access to detailed accounts of the health and social consequences of the disaster. The site also provides a link to international organizations that offer aid to Chernobyl survivors.
www.chernobyl.info

THE NUCLEAR ENERGY INSTITUTE (NEI)

The Nuclear Energy Institute is the policy organization of the nuclear-energy and technologies industry. Its objective is to promote the benefits of nuclear-energy use around the world. The Web site links to information about safety, environmental preservation, and nuclear-waste disposal.
www.nei.org

Index